Crystals: Complete Guide to Crystals

Heal Yourself with Crystals and Healing Stones

Table of Contents

Introduction

Chapter 1: How Crystals Can Aid Healing

Chapter 2: Cleansing, Energizing & Programming

Chapter 3: How to Use Crystals for Healing

Chapter 4: Chakra Crystals

Chapter 5: Crystal, Stone & Mineral Properties

Conclusion and Thank you!

My Other Best Selling Books!

Introduction

I want to thank you and congratulate you for purchasing the book, "Crystals: The Complete Guide to Crystals".

In this book you will learn how to recognize the difference between crystals, stones and some minerals and discover the secrets to healing yourself with crystal energy. You will learn how to cleanse, energize and program stones to work with your body's natural energies.

You will gain knowledge of the seven main Chakras and their importance in the health of your emotional, physical, mental and spiritual well-being. You will learn about the ease with which you can achieve noticeable differences in your general health. Before long you will also be able to guide your family and friends to overall improved well-being.

Thanks again for purchasing this book, I hope you enjoy it!

Chapter 1: How Crystals Can Aid Healing

To many people a crystal is simply a pretty stone, but in truth it is an element which, much like you and me, has been created by nature. It is a natural, organic substance grown over many years from the earth itself. Everything organic to nature contains the universal energies of the universe and are therefore connected to everything else.

We view ourselves as a mind and body, a physical, tangible thing that we can connect with using all of our senses, but we are much more than that. The physical body and all its many attributes is simply an overcoat that we must wear to allow us to interact with the physical world and others in it. Housed within that body is our spirit, a far bigger and stronger entity than what we can see with human eyes. This spirit is pure energy, our life force or chi, and it is connected to all other universal energies.

Why, then, would we assume a stone, crystal, tree, mineral and all other things natural in this world would not also have that energy running through it?

Don't just take my word for it; test this for yourself. Pick up a stone, a pebble or a crystal and calm your mind. Close your eyes and relax and focus only on what you can feel. Focus your mind onto the stone you are holding and feel it. If you have relaxed enough and opened your mind you will feel a pulse coming from the stone. You may sense this as a throbbing, a tingle or even a vibration. This is the universal energy contained with the stone you hold.

The stones/crystals each have different levels of energies that connect with various aspects of the mind and body. Some hold strong levels of energy, others much less, and different stones will emit different levels of energy. Some will be barely noticeable whilst others with give out strong, deep vibrations.

All things natural in this world hold the potential to heal as the energy they contain is able to connect to our own energies and be directed toward specific areas within our physical, mental, emotional, as well as spiritual, selves.

When the energy within us is balanced then we experience health and well-being; unbalanced energies lead to sickness in one form or another. Quite often, this primary imbalance/sickness is the catalyst to all other ailments that we suffer from.

Crystals, gemstones and minerals contain a pure vibration of energy, which then connects and helps to rebalance our own levels.

There are patterns in the energy vibrations and frequencies of nature, and these patterns are consistent in all natural things. By opening up our minds we can allow our own vibrations to stabilize with the vibrations of the stones we wear or come into contact with, in the same way that coming into contact with negative vibrations can unbalance us.

Civilizations have been using the natural energy inherent in the earth to heal and guide us for thousands of years. It is only in the last few centuries that this has become a distant memory and was reduced to 'old wives tales'. Thankfully, many cultures have retained this knowledge and continued to pass it down from generation to generation. Slowly, over the last few decades, a resurgence of interest has occurred in natural healing and more and more people are turning aside from commercial, man-made remedies in favor of exploring all aspects of this fascinating subject.

Science has regularly attempted to diminish the impact of this, but with more people regularly obtaining better results than those who stick to manufactured pharmaceuticals, the impact of natural healing is finally being experienced again. This is not to say that medicines do not have their place in modern day life—they do—but they are not the be all and end all of all things curative.

There are different types of stones and minerals that can be used to heal. Stones and minerals come directly from their formation in the earth whereas crystals are formed from liquids and natural gases. Because of this, a crystal may contain shadows or other crystals that have formed within the primary crystal. Their very structure allows additional attributes to be stored within their structure and this causes them to become electrically charged. This is not a level of natural electricity that is going to give you a shock, but these pockets of energy enable the crystal to alter the energies of other stones and minerals.

A stone or mineral remains that through its lifetime, but when intense levels of pressure or heat are applied to a crystal it can not only alter its shape and form but can, in fact, change it into a completely different type of crystal or mineral.

Using the energy of crystals, stones and minerals is not something that only a few specially gifted people can do; it is accessible to all of us and is inexpensive and simple. All it requires is a small amount of knowledge and practice. Many people who wear jewelry are already experiencing some form of crystal healing, just by being in contact with the stone; they just don't realize it.

Chapter 2: Cleansing, Energizing & Programming

Although crystals, stones and minerals contain pure energy, over time they will absorb the energies of all things they have been exposed to. Stones that have been in contact with anything else containing energy will have taken in the emotions and energies of all who have touched them, so it is essential to always cleanse your crystals regularly. Depending on how often you use them, this may be as frequent as once a week, but judge the regularity based on how often they are handled and used; if using for healing I would recommend they be cleansed before each use.

Cleansing your crystals does not mean scrubbing off any surface dirt with a bowl of soapy water, it means removing all 'stored energy'. If you allow your crystals to be used without cleansing, you risk any stored energies, both negative and positive, being released and transferred. By cleaning it you retain only its natural energies, which can then be used to aid healing.

There are several ways to cleanse your stones, so read through the information below and choose a way that you feel most comfortable with.

Cleansing

There are three methods of salt cleansing: salt water, salt contact and non-contact salt. As some crystals and stones are porous, not all are recommended as the salt can be absorbed and alter the crystal's properties; remember, salt itself is a crystal. Any stone, mineral or crystal that contains water or metal cannot be cleaned using salt water. Any salt can be used; sea salt is the primary choice, but basic kitchen salt is fine. The following should not be cleansed using salt water and you should avoid direct salt contact with all crystals.

Azurite, Beryl, Calcite, Emerald, Garnet, Gypsum, Halite, Hematite, Jet, Lapis Lazuli, Malachite, Moonstone, Opal, Pyrite, Ruby, Sapphire, Selenite, Tanzanite, Tigers Eye, Topaz, Tourmaline, Turquoise.

Salt Water

Fill a bowl (not metal), with water and salt mixture and submerge your stones/minerals. Leave to soak in the salt water for 1 – 24 hours. Ideally, a newly obtained stone should be left for 3 – 7 days to ensure a deep cleansing.

When you remove your stones, hold them under running water to remove any salt residue.

Salt Contact

Fill a bowl with salt and place your stones into it. Stones can be left sitting on the surface of the salt but for a deep, thorough cleansing I recommend you bury them within the salt. Leave for a minimum of 12 hours or for up to 1 week. As with salt water, stones must be rinsed to remove residual salt.

Salt – Non-Contact

This is a great method for any porous crystals, stones or minerals. Fill a bowl with salt. Place a smaller container into the salt. Ensure this is buried between half to three quarters deep. Place your stones into the smaller container. This takes longer to withdraw the stored energies but is just as effective as other salt methods. Leave for 2 to 7 days.

Geode Caves

Geode caves can be expensive to purchase but are highly effective in cleansing crystals. Quartz or Amethyst geodes will absorb all energy from your crystals, neutralize negative energies and then transfer pure energy back into your crystal.

Smudging

Smudging is a method of placing crystals in the smoke from an incense stick. The elements contained within the smoke from the incense will purge the stored energy within the crystal. Light the incense or smudging stick and allow the crystal to be suffused with the smoke for 30 seconds to 1 minute.

Only certain incenses will be effective for this type of cleansing, and the most recommended of these are Cedar wood, Sage and Sandalwood.

Energizing your Crystals

After cleansing, a stone, crystal or mineral will need to be re-energized to ensure it can effectively release its energies. There are three ways to energize your stones.

Water

Running water is the quickest and easiest way to re-energize a stone. The perfect method is to put it into a small mesh bag and place it into a stream. Of course, we are not all lucky enough to live close to natural running water, so an alternative is to place your stone into a glass and leave it under a running tap for 10 – 20 minutes.

Only use water on stones that are not adversely affected by it.

Natural Light

Sunlight or moonlight is a natural way to energize your stones. (Some colored stones may fade when in direct contact with sunlight, so moonlight is the safest option.) Once you have cleansed your crystals, place them in the sunlight or moonlight for 1 – 2 days.

Contact

Many cultures use the body's natural energies to re-energize crystals. Simply hold the stone in your hand for up to 30 minutes.

Personally, while I trust that this is effective, I prefer to use water or moonlight to re-energize my stones.

Programming your Crystals

Crystals do not need to be programmed to work effectively, however, charging your stones for a specific use can be highly beneficial.

Once cleansed and energized, hold the crystal in your hands, close your eyes and relax. Concentrate your thoughts on the specific use you intend for that crystal and visualize the crystal, stone or mineral absorbing your thoughts and energy. The time required to do this varies from person to person, so start with a minimum of 5 minutes of channeling your thoughts and continue until you instinctively feel you have done enough.

You must ensure that your thoughts do not become distracted while you are doing this. Keep your mind solely on the specific use of your stone.

Chapter 3: How to Use Crystals for Healing

There is much versatility in the way crystals, stones and minerals may be used in the practice of healing the mind and body. These range from ways to utilize a stone's energies by placing it on or around you to the directed channeling of the energy using meditation and your Chakras. All forms are effective and it is entirely dependent on your own personal choice which option you prefer to use at any given time. The only consideration should be the objective you are using crystals for and the best way to gain results.

This chapter explores the following techniques:

- Wearing
- Sleeping
- Bathing with Crystals
- Meditation
- Chakra Cleansing

Wearing your Crystals, Stones & Minerals

Whatever way you choose to wear your stones will have some benefit, but the closer they are to the body, the stronger the effect. If your stone is close to a Chakra point then the stone's influence will be strongly directed to the parts of your body and mind that are controlled by that particular Chakra. It will also continue to affect the areas linked with your stone.

When choosing your stones, try to let your unconscious mind direct you to the right stone for you. While all stones will have some benefit, the ones your spirit (intuition) chooses for you will have the strongest impact.

The most common form of wearing a stone is in a piece of jewelry but you can also carry them on your person in a small pouch, place them in a pocket or even sew them into the inside of your clothing. However you choose to wear them, the healing energy will entwine with your own energies and be directed to where they need to be.

Sleeping

Placing a crystal beneath your pillow or close to you on your nightstand will allow you to gain its healing benefits while you sleep.

Some stones have properties which can aid with sleep related problems or the ability to recall your dreams, help with astral sleep travel and ward off bad dreams.

Bathing

Taking a bath is a relaxing, enjoyable and cleansing process on its own; by adding crystals to the mix you can enjoy healing while bathing, too.

Stones, minerals and crystals, with the exception of those stones that suffer adverse affects when wet, can be placed into your bath water, allowing the stone's energies to have direct contact with your body through the water.

Alternately, placing stones around the edge of your bath and in your bathroom will gain you healing benefits while you are bathing. This will be a more subtle energy as it not in direct contact with your own energy fields, but nevertheless, it will be beneficial.

Meditation

Many people who practice meditation will add a crystal or two to their daily meditations. The goal is twofold when meditating; not only will you be using the crystal's energy for healing, you will also be using it to strengthen your protection barriers.

During meditation you can place a crystal on the floor in front of you, wear it or hold it in your hands. While meditating, focus your mind onto the benefits of the crystal and direct your energy into it.

Additional benefits to using crystals while meditating are that many have properties that aid relaxation and focus, two extremely important elements in meditation techniques. It is also very likely that your Chakras have been opened while you are meditating, so the stone's energies can help with cleansing and balancing your Chakra points.

Chakras

Laying relevant stones upon your Chakra points for around 10 minutes per day aids your life force energy to being effectively channeled through your Chakras, clearing any blockages, cleansing the Chakra point and balancing your energies. You can also use this method to direct strong streams of energy to areas of your body that may be healing.

Chapter 4: Chakra Crystals

Your Chakra points are points of energy that is centralized into a particular area of your body. Their main purpose is to allow the flow of your life energy/ universal energy evenly through your body.
Each main point then has several branches that lead from it directly to other areas within your body and mind. Keeping your energy flow regulated and balanced will assist in the overall health of your physical, mental, emotional and spiritual being.

Each Chakra has particular areas which it has influence over, including everything from your psychological and cognitive behaviors, organs, circulation, and hormones to every other mind and body function.

If the flow of your life energy is unbalanced, too quick or too slow, then you will feel it physically and mentally. The more you learn about yourself and your body, the easier it will be for you to recognize if you have blockages within your main Chakras.

There are many Chakras in the human body; most are internal while a few are external to your physical self. The most commonly used Chakras in healing are the seven main energy points which channel energy vertically through the center of your body while feeding all minor energy centers.

First Chakra

The first primary Chakra is situated within the pelvis. It is the 'Root Chakra' and is linked with the color red.

This Chakra governs your survival instinct and physical energy levels. The Root is the base of all physical functions. The natural instinct of self-preservation is born in this Chakra. It is also your grounding Chakra and helps to keep psychological issues in check.

Physical areas controlled by the Root Chakra are the spine, your hormone-producing adrenal glands, the bladder and prostate, and your kidneys.

If this Chakra becomes blocked you may begin to suffer with psychological disturbances, which can cause aggressive thoughts and actions, sexual dysfunction such as impotency, a lack of self-belief along with panic and anxiety attacks, hypertension, eating disorders and depression.

Stones associated with this chakra are:

- Obsidian
- Black Tourmaline
- Garnet
- Ruby

- Smoky Quartz

- Hematite

- All other red or black stones, crystals or minerals

Second Chakra

The Sacral Chakra is situated between your navel and your pelvis and is associated with the color orange. This is your pleasure Chakra and controls all forms of creativity.

It is also responsible for reproduction and sexual energy, legs and the reproductive organs. When it becomes blocked your imagination and creativity are stifled, leading to problems with depression, sexual pleasure addiction and other dependent behaviors and irrational thoughts and actions.

Physically you will begin to experience signs of urinary problems, kidney issues, bowel upsets and back problems as well as hormonal disruptions, which can cause infertility.

Stones associated with this chakra are:

- Blue Turquoise

- Blue Fluorite

- Orange Calcite

- Carnelian

- All other blue/green and orange stones

Third Chakra

The Solar Plexus Chakra is located around the Navel and is associated with the color Yellow. This is the Chakra that controls our intelligence and recognition of the sense of who we truly are.

When balanced, this energy center aids us in the knowledge of what we want to do, what we need, self-control, confidence and a balanced control of our thoughts and actions.

It is also aligned with the liver, stomach, gall bladder and pancreas, and when blocked it can lead to problems with weight gain, diabetes, respiratory issues, digestion problems, stomach ulcers and pain in our nerve endings.

It also affects anxiety levels and produces a need to control others in the attempt to gain control of ourselves. Self-doubt and insecurity can manifest and very little action follows from the plans we make.

Stones associated with this Chakra are:

- Citrine
- Yellow Jasper
- Yellow Topaz
- Pyrite

- All other yellow/gold stones

Fourth Chakra

This Chakra is located slightly to the right of your heart, in the center of your chest, and is linked with the color green. The Heart Chakra is also the gateway to our inner spirit and is linked to your emotions.

Everything from compassion, empathy, unconditional love, peace and happiness are connected to this Chakra. It is also responsible for circulation, the heart, lungs and the liver.

When this becomes blocked, social situations become difficult and social anxiety and a mistrust of other people begin to develop. Judgment of others becomes confused and a retreat into isolation starts to occur.

Additionally, symptoms of bad circulation and respiratory problems begin to increase and panic attacks are often suffered.

Stones associated with this Chakra are:

- Rose Quartz

- Pink Tourmaline

- Malachite

- Jade

- And all other green or pink stones

Fifth Chakra

Your fifth main Chakra is the Throat Chakra and it is linked with the color blue. This is the Chakra that relates to all aspects of communication, intellect, integrity and expression of self. It also governs the lungs, the thyroid gland, digestion, upper arms and all aspects of the throat.

If this Chakra becomes blocked many of the symptoms of a blocked Heart Chakra begin to manifest along with problems communicating with others and erratic and unstable behavior.

Head pain, thyroid issues, pain in the neck area, gingivitis, laryngitis, ulcers and all throat problems are also common with a blocked Throat Chakra.

Stones associated with this Chakra are:

- Sapphire
- Blue Calcite
- Blue Beryl
- Blue Tourmaline
- All other blue colored stones

Sixth Chakra

This is the Third Eye Chakra and it is located in the forehead, centralized between the eyebrows. Its color is Indigo and it is the center of our spiritual vision and linked to our imagination.

It also governs the pituitary gland, the lower brain, the spinal column, the left eye and our ears and nose. This is the gateway to the realm of spiritualism and psychic ability.

Issues with the sciatic nerve are quite common when this Chakra is blocked, along with migraines, sinus problems, the possibility of seizures and eyesight problems developing or worsening.

Psychological abilities become problematic with anxiety disorders and depression often manifesting alongside paranoid thoughts and delusions.

Stones associated with this Chakra are:

- Lapis Lazuli

- Azurite

- Sodalite

- Flourite

- All other Indigo colored stones

Seventh Chakra

The Crown Chakra is purple but is also depicted as white in many teachings. It is situated at the crown of the head, near the pineal gland. This is the gateway to the center of our true being and gives us access to wisdom and total spiritual awareness. It is also the control center for the pineal gland, upper brain and the right eye.

A blocked Crown Chakra causes a development of disconnection with others, mentally, physically and emotionally. This is primarily because we are disconnected with ourselves, which leads us to an inability to form connections with others. We feel isolated and lack true understanding of anything around us, causing delusions, headache, cognitive disruption, insomnia and depression. We stop being able to plan and think beyond the here and now, which causes a vicious circle of the need to connect, to the inability to follow through on the connections, to isolation, depression and insomnia.

Stones associated with this Chakra are:

- Amethyst

- White Calcite

- Alexandrite

- Opal

- Purple Opal

- All other purple and white stones

In addition to these specific stones, clear quartz can be used on any or all of the Chakra points.

Chapter 5: Crystal, Stone & Mineral Properties

Agate

There are many forms of Agate that vary in style and color, with the majority containing bands running through them, although some forms contain markings that resemble leaves and other vegetation. It is a type of Chalcedony and is formed predominantly in volcanic rock. Agate is helpful in removing fears, creating peace and harmony, enhancing confidence and giving strength and energy. It is also useful in stimulating intellectual thought and creativity. It is also believed to assist in the healing of gum and mouth problems.

Amazonite

A green/aqua colored stone, Amazonite is the stone of communication, truth, loyalty and trust. It aids in the development of psychic ability, creativity, intelligence and intuition. It aids in calming the ego and promoting feelings of self-esteem by reducing stress and negative psychological thought processes. All emotional disruptions begin to calm with the use of Amazonite. It is also a useful stone for reducing nervous dispositions, aiding the healing of bone, teeth and nails and lowering the heart rate.

Amber

Despite its appearance, Amber is not actually a stone, crystal or mineral; it is petrified tree sap from the pine tree and each piece can date back up to a million years. Quite often amber contains prehistoric fossils from insects, seeds, leaves, flowers and all manner of natural debris.

Amber has absorbing energies that draw illness and disease from the body. It absorbs pain and negativity and helps to ground the mind. It is also a strong stone for strengthening the muscles that produce mucus and those of the mind, helping to improve your emotional and intellectual abilities along with your memory.

Throat and stomach issues can be improved with Amber along with any symptoms relating to the blood, bladder, kidneys, liver, throat, bones, skin and eyes. Stress is calmed and all symptoms that stem from it begin to abate.

Amethyst

Amethyst is reputed to be the stone of sobriety and as such, aids with healing alcoholism and all other types of addictions. It stabilizes energy and promotes feelings of courage, calmness, inner strength and balance. It is reputed to protect against psychic attack and aids psychic ability. Amethyst also helps with communication and promotes happiness, calms headaches, arthritis and other general pain, eases symptoms of fibromyalgia and chronic fatigue along with boosting the immune system.

Aventurine – Blue

Blue Aventurine calms and stabilizes the emotions and aids with communication and creativity. It has positive benefits on all elements of the Throat Chakra and enhances the intuition.

Aventurine – Green

Green Aventurine promotes a positive outlook and strengthens the imagination. It is also useful in problems concerning the circulatory system, issues with sleep and headaches.

Aventurine – Orange

Orange Aventurine gently breaks down symptoms that have occurred following sexual trauma and helps to strengthen all areas of communication and intellect. It works well in stimulating increased feelings of self-worth and the imagination.

Aquamarine

Aquamarine is the courage stone. It allows creativity and communication to flow well by stimulating confidence levels and calming the mind. All symptoms relating to mental health are eased and intuition increases, along with benefits relating to all aspects of the Heart and Throat Chakras.

Beryl

Beryl comes in a variety of colors with shades of green, yellow, blue, pink and white, and is an extremely helpful stone in dealing with stress and the symptoms that result from it. It calms anxiety and quiets an over-stimulated mind.

It aids recovery of problems with the liver, stomach, spleen and the circulatory and pulmonary systems as well as aiding the body with detoxification.

Black Tourmaline

Black tourmaline is a good stone for grounding excess nervous energy through its use in transforming negative energies into positive energy. Obsessive behavior is tempered, fears calmed and psychological/emotional energy is balanced with Black Tourmaline. It also strengthens the immune system and aids healing in arthritis and heart problems.

Bloodstone

A stone of courage, Bloodstone helps to relieve depressive illnesses and anxiety, promotes energy levels as well as detoxifies the system. It is extremely effective in strengthening the mind when in stressful situations and improves clarity of thought while revitalizing the mind and body.

Bloodstone is reputed to be able to ward off the effects of colds, the flu, inflammations and infection.

Blue Quartz

Blue Quartz helps the mind to think with clarity and organizes thoughts. It strengthens self-discipline and boosts creativity and expression of self, stimulating your courage and weakening the mind's hold on fears.

All aspects of the third eye chakra benefit from this crystal along with a reduction in hyperactivity caused by overstimulation, healing for the thyroid, spleen, throat and endocrine system.

Carnelian

Carnelian is a creative stone of the agate family. It helps to relieve emotions and tension caused by them and promotes a sense of courage and individuality.

This is a rejuvenating stone that will help with rheumatism and colds, hay fever, kidney stones and promote healing of the skin.

Carnelian will strengthen all the areas governed by both the Root Chakra and the Sacral Chakra.

Citrine

Citrine is most beneficial to the areas of the body and mind associated with the Solar Plexus Chakra, but it is equally effective in treating a lack of self-belief and strengthening willpower.

It is a stone which promotes happiness and eases depression, irrational thought processes and mood swings along with promoting healing of the digestive system.

Clear Quartz

Clear Quart is a wonder stone that aids healing in most areas. It is a good general purpose healing crystal that helps to create a balance within the life force energy.

It is directly linked with the Crown Chakra and all things related to it but will cleanse negativity and aid the healing of all Chakra points.

Emerald

Emerald is another good stone for all general healing but is particular useful for the respiratory system, heart, circulatory system, pancreas, thymus and eyesight. It also gives strength to the spine and helps to detoxify the body and improve the immune system.

Spiritually the emerald helps to raise consciousness and can be extremely effective as a tool when meditating. It also strengthens the aura.

Garnet

Garnet is a cleanser of the Chakras, balancing the energy and rejuvenating the system. If you are looking to increase your sex drive then garnet is the stone to use and will also create emotional calm.

This stone will add strength to all aspects of the Root Chakra and the Heart Chakra and will increase your perceptions of others, helping to remove inhibition and increase self-confidence.

Physically garnet will aid in bringing relief to symptoms relating to the blood, heart, respiratory system, spine and bone, along with strengthening the immune system. This is also a useful stone to use to calm any issues of excess anger.

Hematite

Hematite is a mind stone promoting clarity of thought, logical thinking and problem solving. It is a grounding stone that helps to balance the energy flow of the body and mind.

Hematite is also known to help lower body temperature, aid with disorders of the blood, promote restful sleep and settle any problems related to the nervous system.

Linked with the Root Chakra, this stone balances all areas connected to it.

Jade

Jade stones help to calm and balance personality traits while relaxing the mind and removing negative thoughts. Become of the calmness it creates, jade helps with the emotional release of pent up feelings and eases the physical symptoms that come from them. Despite its calming effect, jade stimulates your creativity and aids in relieving irritability so new ideas can form.

In some cultures, jade is referred to as a dream stone as it frees the mind to experience dreams of insight and promotes a sense of being true to who you are. Jade is detoxifying and adds healing to the kidneys and adrenal glands. It is also useful for fertility problems and takes care of bones.

Lapis Lazuli

Lapis Lazuli is a versatile stone that influences communication, kidney function and hormones. It promotes a feeling of comfort when speaking freely and helps to ground the body and mind. It stimulates the thyroid and kidneys, helping to rid the body of toxins while aiding in the dissipation of fat tissue.

This stone is ideal for any ladies who suffer with erratic hormone levels as it balances the adrenal gland, helping to produce a stabilized level of hormone release.

Lapis is linked to both the Throat Chakra and the Third Eye Chakra and works to aid the link between the conscious world and the external universal energies.

Orange Calcite

Orange Calcite increases confidence and creative thoughts and focus, stimulating the imagination and providing strength to fulfill any plans you make.

Use of this stone promotes a lift in mood and can help with shyness, depression and a stifled sex drive.

Its main area of healing is the clearing of any blockages within the Solar Plexus and Sacral Chakras.

Peridot

Negative emotional states are eased with peridot and the nervous system is calmed. It promotes healing with all emotional issues and their symptoms and adds additional strength to the body's healing abilities.

Pyrite

Pyrite, better known as fool's gold, is an intelligence stone that enhances mental abilities including logic, creativity and imagination, psychic ability, memory, psychological balance and intelligence.

Red Jasper

Red Jasper balances and stabilizes the life force energy allowing it to flow in a slow and steady stream. This ability to balance energy helps the mind to stay calm and in control.

This stone is linked to the Root and Sacral Chakras and will have a positive effect on all areas that are associated with them.

Rose Quartz

Rose Quartz is the stone of love and is linked with the Heart Chakra, affecting a positive change to all things this Chakra controls. It brings a calm serenity and a general feeling of happiness and well-being.

Smoky Quartz

Smoky Quartz is a crystal that will aid in the relieving of depressive feelings and emotions along with all symptoms that result from this. It removes negative energy and grounds the mind, providing access to the knowledge hidden in the subconscious.

Linked to the Root Chakra, this crystal aids the healing of the abdomen, reproductive system, hormonal imbalance, kidneys and pancreas and relieves water retention.

Sodalite

The stone of rational thought and cognitive reasoning, sodalite helps with communication problems and is a stimulant for thought processing. It aids focus, increasing the ability to learn and retain knowledge.

Sodalite also heals the digestive system, promotes a restful sleep by relieving insomnia issues and is useful in the speeding the recovery from colds and flu. This stone is linked to both the Third Eye Chakra and the Throat Chakra.

Tigers Eye

Tigers Eye is focused on grounding which helps with practical thinking, clear mental vision and strength of will. It is linked with the Solar Plexus Chakra and affects all mental, physical and emotional abilities relating to this Chakra.

Tourmaline

Tourmaline comes in a variety of colors, and all enhance the mood and promote inner confidence and calm and aid the lymphatic system.

- Blue Tourmalines works with throat and thyroid issues and enhances speech. It also reduces mental tension.

- Pink Tourmaline aids with balance of the emotions and promotes a greater understanding of who you are and how you feel. It guides the transformation of negativity into positivity and calms and strengthens the mind.

- Black and Green Tourmaline help to regulate blood pressure and reduce stresses of the nervous system.

Turquoise

Turquoise provides healing for the entire body and mind. It helps heal the respiratory system and strengthens communication and the immune system.

Turquoise is linked to all aspects of both the Heart and Throat Chakras and strengthens the link between the Chakras.

Conclusion

I hope this book was able to help you to understand the healing benefits of crystals and how easy they are to use, and that it has given you the confidence to try crystal healing for yourself!

Finally, if you enjoyed this book, then I'd like to ask you for a favor. Would you be kind enough to leave a review for this book on Amazon? It really helps me out and is greatly appreciated!

Thank you and good luck!

Here Are My Other Best Selling Books On Amazon!

Below you'll find some of my other best selling books on Amazon and Kindle as well.

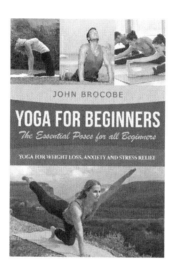

Yoga for Beginners: The Essential Poses for All Beginners, with Pictures:

Go to: amzn.to/1VC8cSv

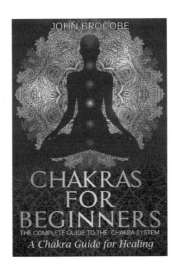

Chakras for Beginners: The Complete Guide to the Chakra System

Go to: amzn.to/1SIvGpu

Made in the USA
Columbia, SC
08 December 2021

50746854R00026